THE

SOUTH BEACH DIET

COOKBOOK

FOR

NEWBIES AND BEGINNERS

BY

Dr. Christen Zimmermann

Table of Contents

INTRODUCTION

Could this low-carb diet give you an edge in losing weight? Help you keep weight off permanently? Here's what you need to know.

 The South Beach Diet is a popular commercial weight-loss diet created in 2003 by cardiologist Arthur Agatston, M.D., and first outlined in the best-selling book "The South Beach Diet: The Delicious, Doctor-Designed, Foolproof Plan for Fast and Healthy Weight Loss."

The South Beach Diet, which is named after a glamorous area of Miami, is sometimes called a modified low-carbohydrate diet. The South Beach Diet is lower in carbs (carbohydrates) and higher in protein and healthy fats than is a typical eating plan. But it's not a strict low-carb diet.

There is also a keto (ketogenic) version of the South Beach diet. Ketogenic diets include very few carbs. The goal of a ketogenic diet is to force the body to use fat for energy instead of carbohydrates or protein.

Purpose

The purpose of the South Beach Diet is to change the overall balance of the foods you eat to encourage weight loss and a healthy lifestyle. The South Beach Diet says it's a healthy way of eating whether you want to lose weight or not.

WHY YOU MIGHT FOLLOW THE SOUTH BEACH DIET

You might choose to follow the South Beach Diet because you:

• Enjoy the types and amounts of food featured in the diet

• Want a diet that restricts certain carbs and fats to help you lose weight

• Want to change your overall eating habits

• Want a diet you can stick with for life

• Like the related South Beach Diet products, such as cookbooks and diet foods

Check with your doctor or dietitian before starting any weight-loss diet, especially if you have any health concerns.

The South Beach Diet says that its balance of complex carbs, lean protein and healthy fats makes it a nutrient-dense, fiber-rich diet that you can follow for a lifetime of healthy eating. Food sources of complex carbs, or so-called good carbs, include fruit, vegetables, whole grains, beans and legumes. Simple carbs, or "bad" carbs, include sugar, syrup and baked goods made from refined white flour.

The South Beach Diet also teaches you about the different kinds of dietary fats and encourages you to limit unhealthy fats while eating more foods with healthier monounsaturated fats. The South Beach Diet emphasizes the benefits of fiber and whole grains and encourages you to include fruits and vegetables in your eating plan.

CARBOHYDRATES

The South Beach Diet is lower in carbohydrates than is a typical eating plan, but not as low as a strict low-carb diet. On a typical eating plan, about 45% to 65% of your daily calories come from carbohydrates. Based on a 2,000-

calorie-a-day diet, this amounts to about 225 to 325 grams of carbohydrates a day.

In the final maintenance phase of the South Beach Diet, you can get as much as 28% of your daily calories from carbohydrates, or about 140 grams of carbohydrates a day. A strict low-carb diet might restrict your carb intake to as little as 20 to 100 grams a day. The keto version of the South Beach diet limits carbs to 40 grams a day during phase 1, and 50 grams during phase 2.

EXERCISE

The South Beach Diet has evolved over time and now recommends exercise as an important part of your lifestyle. The South Beach Diet says that regular exercise will boost your metabolism and help prevent weight-loss plateaus.

Here are our favorite South Beach Diet recipes to try this year. These low-carb, low-sugar and high protein recipes are also delicious, healthy and easy to prepare.

SHRIMP SCAMPI WITH ZOODLES

Cook up a classic with a low-carb twist! Zucchini noodles are the perfect pasta replacement in this simple Shrimp Scampi With Zoodles. Minced garlic, spicy red pepper flakes, savory chicken broth and zesty lemon juice add big flavor and brightness to the rich, buttery sauce. While the flavor is out of this world, the best part about this dish is definitely the simplicity. Because it's ready for the dinner table in only a few short minutes, you can whip up this pasta dinner with minimal effort after a long, busy day.

Ingredients:

• 2 Tbsp. unsalted butter

• 1 lb. tail-on large shrimp, peeled and deveined

• 4 cloves garlic, minced

• ½ teaspoon red pepper flakes

• ¼ cup low sodium chicken broth

• Juice of 1 lemon

• 1 ½ lb. zucchini noodles

• 2 Tbsp. grated Parmesan cheese

• 2 Tbsp. fresh parsley, chopped

Directions:

• Melt butter in a large skillet over medium-high heat. Add the shrimp, garlic and red pepper flakes. Season with salt and pepper to taste. Cook the shrimp for 2-3 minutes per side, until shrimp are pink.

• Transfer the shrimp to a plate and set aside. Add broth and lemon juice to the pan. Bring to a simmer. Stir in zucchini noodles and return shrimp to pan. Cook 1-2 minutes, until zucchini is crisp-tender. Top with Parmesan cheese and fresh parsley before serving.

I dip, you dip, we dip. Who doesn't love a delicious dip? We sure do, and this is one of our favorites. Our Creamy Avocado Pesto Dip is packed with flavor and South Beach-approved.

Ingredients:

• 1/3 cup pine nuts

• 1 large bunch basil

• 1 garlic clove, peeled

• 1/4 cup avocado oil

• 3 Tbsp. avocado

• 2 tsp. lemon juice

• 1/4 tsp. sea salt

Directions:

1. Heat oven or toaster to 275°F. Spread pine nuts on a baking tray and bake until fragrant and lightly browned, about 10 minutes. Cool slightly, about 3 minutes.

2. Add the basil, garlic and pine nuts to a food processor and pulse until coarsely chopped.

3. With the food processor running, add the avocado oil in a steady stream.

4. Add fresh avocado, lemon juice and salt. Pulse a few times to combine and serve.

There is no better start to the day than waking up to a stack of warm flapjacks. Try these low-carb Peanut Butter Pancakes made with a nutrient-rich zucchini and almond flour base.

Ingredients:

• ½ cup creamy, natural peanut butter (no sugar added)

• 4 eggs

• 1 cup zucchini, diced

• ¼ tsp. salt

• ½ tsp. baking powder

• 2 tsp. stevia

• 1 tsp. vanilla extract

• 1 tsp. cinnamon

• ½ cup almond flour

Directions:

1. Place all ingredients into a blender and blend until smooth.

2. Preheat a large pan over medium heat and spray with nonstick cooking spray.

3. Using a ¼ cup measuring cup, pour the batter into the pan to create pancakes.

4. Cook the pancakes until bubbles start to form on the batter, about 2-3 minutes. Carefully flip using a spatula and continue to cook for another minute.

5. Repeat steps 3 & 4 until all the batter is used.

6. Serve with desired toppings.

Cauliflower Walnut Taco Meat

This meatless taco meat has an undeniably crumbly, meaty texture and is the perfect plant-based addition to tacos, burrito bowls and salads. Even better, this healthy recipe is vegan, gluten free and low carb! Add it to all of your favorite meals for a spicy and satisfying supper.

Ingredients:

• 4 cups cauliflower florets

• 1 cup walnuts

• 1 Tbsp. olive oil

• 1 ¼ tsp. salt

• 1 Tbsp. cumin

• 1 Tbsp. smoked paprika

• 1 tsp. garlic powder

• 1 tsp. onion powder

• 1 Tbsp. tomato paste

• 1 Tbsp. Dijon mustard

• 1-2 tsp. hot sauce (optional)

Directions:

1. Pulse cauliflower and walnuts in a food processor until broken down into small, pea-sized pieces. Heat olive oil in a large pan over medium-high heat. Add cauliflower-walnut mixture and cook for 5-6 minutes, or until cauliflower is cooked through, stirring occasionally.

2. Add all remaining ingredients to the pan and stir well to coat. Cook another 2-3 minutes, or until mixture is crumbly and resembles taco meat. Season with salt and pepper to taste. Use in any recipe that calls for taco meat, including but not limited to tacos, lettuce wraps, chili, quesadillas, burrito bowls, salads, casseroles, pizza, etc.

Avocado Crab Salad

Creamy avocado and sweet lump crab meat are piled atop a bed of fresh green lettuce. Get the recipe for this simple Avocado Crab Salad.

Ingredients:

- 8 oz. lump crab meat

- ½ cup plum or roma tomato, seeded and diced

- 2 Tbsp. red onion, diced fine

- 1 avocado, seeded and diced

- 3 Tbsp. mayonnaise

- 2 tsp. Old Bay seasoning

- 2 Tbsp lemon juice

- 1 cup green leaf lettuce

Directions:

1. Prepare the lump crab meat by draining and ensuring no soft shells remain if needed.

2. Mix together crab, tomatoes, onions, mayonnaise, seasoning and lemon juice. You can either mix in the avocado or serve it separately on the side.

3. Arrange green leaf lettuce on three bowls or plates. Top each with 1/3 of the crab mixture.

4. Serve with a wedge of lemon.

Ingredients:

• Pesto

• 1 head endive, washed and trimmed

• 1 small head garlic

• 3 Tbsp. olive oil, divided

• 1/2 cup mint, packed

• 1/4 cup grated Parmesan

• 1/3 cup ground walnuts

• 1 lemon, juiced and zested

• Salmon Cakes

• 3/4 lb. boneless skinless salmon, cooked

• 1 cup cauliflower, cooked

• 1 large egg, lightly beaten

• 1 Tbsp. mayonnaise, no sugar added

• 1 Tbsp. dill, finely chopped

- 2 Tbsp. flat leaf parsley, finely chopped

- 1/2 cup almond meal

- 1 Tbsp. olive oil

- 1/3 cup shredded sharp cheddar cheese (optional)

- To Serve

- Lemon wedges

- 1 large handful baby arugula or watercress

Directions:

1. Preheat the oven to 425°F.

2. To make the pesto, slice endive in half lengthwise and place in a small baking dish. Season with salt and pepper to taste, then drizzle with 1/2 tablespoon of olive oil. Set aside.

3. Slice the top off of the garlic head to expose cloves. Brush with 1/2 tablespoon of olive oil, then wrap tightly in aluminum foil. Place in a small baking dish and transfer to oven. Cook 35 to 45 minutes.

4. When the garlic has been cooking for 20 minutes, transfer baking dish with endive to the oven and bake 25 minutes, until golden.

5. Transfer the roasted endive and garlic to a blender. Add remaining 2 tablespoons of olive oil, mint, Parmesan, walnuts, lemon juice, lemon zest, and salt and pepper to taste. Process until creamy.

6. Line a baking sheet with parchment paper. Set aside.

7. To make the salmon cakes, flake the salmon and add it to a large bowl with cauliflower, egg, mayonnaise, dill, parsley, and salt and pepper to taste. Mix well to combine.

8. Add 1/4 cup of almond meal to the salmon mixture and stir to combine.

9. Form the mixture into 8 patties. If the mixture is too loose, transfer it to the refrigerator for 15 minutes until it firms up. Roll the patties in the remaining almond meal. Place on the prepared baking sheet.

10. Brush the patties with olive oil and sprinkle with some cheddar cheese (optional). Bake 12 to 15 minutes, flipping halfway through, until crisp and golden.

11. Serve with lemon wedges and arugula.

Spring has arrived! Celebrate the season of warm weather, sunshine and blooming flowers with a fresh and fun recipe filled with crunchy veggies, crispy bacon and creamy dressing. This low-carb Layered Salad is to easy make and easy to enjoy!

Ingredients:

• 8 cups romaine and iceberg lettuce, torn into bite-sized pieces

• ½ red onion, thinly sliced

• 10 oz. frozen green peas

• ¾ cup celery, chopped

• 1 cup shredded cheddar cheese, divided

• 1 cup broccoli, blanched for 2 minutes in boiling water

• 1 2.25-oz. can sliced black olives

• 1 lb. cooked and crumbled bacon, divided

• Dressing

• ¾ cup light mayonnaise

• ¾ cup light sour cream

Directions:

1. Using a 9 x 13 glass dish, layer the ingredients in the following order: lettuce, onion, green peas, celery, ¾ cup of the cheese, broccoli, olives and ¾ of the bacon.

2. Mix together the dressing ingredients in a small bowl.

3. Pour the dressing over the salad. Carefully spread it evenly with a spatula.

4. Top salad with the remaining cheese and bacon.

5. Cover and refrigerate overnight for at least 8 hours, preferably overnight.

If you're craving hot wings but don't want to damage your weight loss success, not to worry. These Buffalo Chicken Zucchini Boats are the perfect replacement. Featuring shredded chicken breast, healthy homemade buffalo sauce, melty cheddar cheese, crunchy celery and even some crispy bacon, it's the ultimate meal that fits into your healthy diet.

Ingredients:

• 12 oz. boneless skinless chicken breasts

• 4 medium zucchini

• 4 slices raw bacon, chopped

• 2 Tbsp. butter

• 2 oz. full-fat cream cheese

• ¼ cup plain whole-milk Greek yogurt

• ¼ cup hot sauce

• ¼ cup chopped celery

• ½ cup shredded full-fat cheddar cheese, divided

• 2 tablespoons chopped fresh cilantro

Directions:

1. Preheat the oven to 375°F.

2. Place the chicken breasts in a medium pot, season with salt, pepper, and a few springs of fresh herbs, and then cover with water. Bring them to a boil over high heat. Reduce the heat to medium and cook for 15 to 20 minutes, until the chicken is cooked through. Remove the chicken breasts from the water, allow to them cool, then shred.

3. Slice the zucchini lengthwise. Scoop out and discard the seeds. Place the zucchini boats side by side in a 9 x 13-inch baking dish.

4. Place the chopped bacon in a medium pot over medium heat. Cook for 5 to 7 minutes, stirring occasionally, until crisp. Remove the bacon to a plate lined with a paper towel and set aside, reserving the bacon grease in the pot.

5. Add the butter to the bacon grease and melt over medium heat. Add the cream cheese, yogurt, and hot sauce. Stir for 1 to 2 minutes, until combined.

6. Remove the sauce from the heat. Add to the sauce the shredded chicken, celery, half the cheddar, and the black beans (if using). Season with salt and pepper to taste. Toss to coat.

7. Divide the chicken mixture evenly among the 8 scooped-out zucchini boats. Sprinkle each boat with the remaining cheddar.

8. Bake for 20 to 22 minutes, until the zucchini is just tender and the cheese is melted.

9. Garnish with the bacon bits and cilantro. Serve warm.

Beef Stroganoff is a simple yet decadent dish that can easily be transformed into a low-carb feast. While a traditional stroganoff is typically served over rice or pasta, we keep our version low-carb and stick to just the beef, cream and veggies. Hearty beef dinners are a staple in your weight loss menu. Stay on plan and prepare a meal that the whole family will love with classic flavors and simple ingredients.

Ingredients:

• 2 Tbsp. olive oil

• 1 lb. steak, cut in 1-inch pieces

• 1 yellow onion, diced

• 1 clove garlic, minced

• 8 oz. container white or baby bella mushrooms, sliced

• 1 cup beef broth

• 1 cup heavy cream

• ½ cup sour cream

• ¼ cup fresh parsley, roughly chopped

• Salt and pepper to taste

Directions:

1. Add the olive oil to a large pan over medium heat. Add the steak cubes to the pan and sauté for about 1 minute on each side or until lightly browned. Remove the steak from the pan and set aside on a plate.

2. Using the same pan, sauté the onions, mushrooms and garlic until cooked and onions are transluscent, about 5 minutes. Add the steak back to the skillet. Add beef broth and heavy cream to the pan and bring to a boil.

3. Turn the heat down and simmer until the steak becomes tender, about 15 minutes. Stir in the sour cream and season with salt and pepper. Garnish with parsley and serve.

Pizza for breakfast is underrated. With its crispy crust, hearty toppings and melty cheese, it seems there is no better way to start the day. We put a morning time spin on this Italian classic by swapping out your average toppings with scrambled eggs, crumbled bacon and shredded cheddar cheese. It's got all the delicious flavors of your favorite breakfast sandwich combined with a nutritious, almond flour-based naan crust. Enjoy your pie under the morning sky with this unique, low carb recipe!

Ingredients:

• ½ cup almond flour

• ½ cup tapioca flour

• 2 tsp. baking powder

• 2 tsp. dried rosemary

• 1 cup whole buttermilk, divided

• 4 slices bacon

• 1 Tbsp. butter

• 6 eggs

• ¾ cup shredded cheddar cheese

Directions:

1. Preheat oven to 400°F.

2. Line a Quarter sheet pan or 9x13 baking dish with parchment paper. Set aside.

3. Sift almond flour, tapioca flour and baking powder into a large mixing bowl.

4. Add rosemary and ¾ cup buttermilk. Whisk until combined.

5. Pour batter onto prepared sheet pan. Transfer pan to oven and bake 12 to 15 minutes, until golden. Remove from oven and poke holes all over naan bread with the tip of a fork. Set aside and keep oven on.

6. Heat bacon in a skillet over medium high. Cook 7-8 minutes, flipping halfway through, until crisp. Remove and set aside.

7. Whisk eggs and remaining buttermilk in a medium mixing bowl.

8. Add butter to skillet used for bacon over medium heat.

9. Add egg mixture to skillet and cook 4 to 5 minutes, until just set, stirring occasionally. Season with salt and pepper to taste.

10. Spread scrambled eggs over naan bread. Crumble bacon on top then sprinkle with cheese.

11. Return sheet pan to oven for 3 to 4 minutes, until cheese is melted.

12. Slice into 6 pieces and enjoy warm.

Beef up your weight loss menu with this easy Beef Burrito Bowl! Featuring perfectly seasoned, smoky ground beef and an array of classic burrito ingredients, this low-carb creation is a must for your meal prep menu.

Ingredients:

• For the Beef

• 1 lb. ground beef

• 2 ½ Tbsp. chili powder

• 1 tsp. ground cumin

• ½ tsp. smoked paprika

• 1 tsp. onion powder

• 1 tsp. garlic powder

• ¼ tsp. sea salt

• ¼ tsp. ground black pepper

• For the Bowls

• 2 tsp. avocado oil

- 4 cups cauliflower rice (1 medium head, grated or finely chopped)

- 1 red onion, diced

- 1 head romaine lettuce, chopped

- ½ cup cherry tomatoes, halved

- 1 cup salsa

- 1 avocado, sliced

- ¼ cup fresh cilantro, chopped

- 1 lime, sliced

Directions:

1. Heat a large skillet over medium-high heat and add the beef. Cook for 2 to 3 minutes, until no longer pink.

2. Add the chili powder, cumin, smoked paprika, onion powder, garlic powder, salt, and pepper. Continue to cook, stirring frequently, until the beef is fully browned, about 5 minutes.

3. In a separate skillet, heat the avocado oil over medium heat and add the cauliflower rice. Cook until tender, about 5 minutes.

4. Assemble 4 bowls with equally distributed cauliflower rice and beef, adding the red onion, lettuce, cherry tomatoes, salsa, avocado, and cilantro. Serve with the lime slices. If you are making this dish ahead of time, leave off the salsa, avocado, cilantro, lettuce, and lime slices until you are ready to eat.

Lamb chops get a slightly sweet spin thanks to the addition of a delicious homemade mint pesto sauce. Add this hearty dish to your St. Patrick's Day menu for a low-carb dinner that the whole family will love.

Ingredients:

• Mint Pesto

• 2/3 cup packed fresh mint leaves

• 1/4 cup packed fresh parsley leaves

• 2 Tbsp. pine nuts or chopped walnuts

• 1 garlic clove, smashed and peeled

• 1/2 tsp. grated lemon zest

• 1 Tbsp. fresh lemon juice

• 1 Tbsp. extra-virgin olive oil

• Lamb Chops

• 8 loin lamb chops (each about 1 inch thick), well trimmed

• Salt and freshly ground black pepper, to taste

Directions:

1. Heat the broiler.

2. For the pesto: In a blender or food processor, process the mint, parsley, nuts, garlic, lemon zest, and lemon juice until finely chopped. With the machine running, drizzle in the oil and process until almost smooth.

3. For the lamb: Place the chops on a broiler pan. Season lightly with salt and pepper. Broil the chops for 3 minutes per side for medium-rare.

4. Transfer 2 chops to each of 4 plates and top evenly with the pesto.

13. Cucumber Feta Salad

Warm weather and sunshine calls for cool, refreshing and hydrating recipes like our low carb Cucumber Feta Salad. This simple side features crunchy cucumbers and creamy feta cheese, all tossed in a homemade Greek-inspired vinaigrette. Serve it up with burgers, grilled meats or salmon for the perfect spring or summer veggie side dish.

Ingredients:

• 1 large seedless cucumber, thinly sliced

• 4 oz. feta cheese, diced into ½ inch cubes

• Dressing

• 1 Tbsp. olive oil

• 1 Tbsp. red wine vinegar

• ¼ tsp. garlic powder

• ¼ tsp. dried oregano

• Salt and pepper, to taste

Directions:

1. Whisk together the dressing ingredients in a large bowl.

2. Add the cucumber and feta cheese. Toss gently to coat in the dressing.

Cold weather calls for soup! This creamy, dreamy broccoli soup is perfect for your fall and winter menu. Fresh broccoli florets are the star of the show, while Greek yogurt, whole milk and chicken broth add a savory flavor and decadent texture. Whip up this low carb soup recipe for the ultimate diet-friendly dish.

Ingredients:

• 6 slices raw bacon, chopped

• 2 Tbsp. butter

• 2 cups broccoli florets

• ¼ cup chopped shallots

• 1 tablespoon minced garlic

• ½ cup plain whole-milk Greek yogurt

• 1 cup whole milk

• 2 cups chicken broth

• 2 Tbsp. lemon juice

• 2 Tbsp. chopped chives

• ¼ cup sliced almonds

Directions:

1. In a large stockpot, heat the chopped bacon over medium heat for 5 to 7 minutes, cooking until crisp. Remove the bacon and set aside, reserving the grease in the pan.

2. Add the butter to the bacon grease and melt.

3. Add the broccoli florets and cook for 4 to 5 minutes, until browned. Add the shallots and garlic and cook for 1 minute, until fragrant.

4. Add the yogurt, whole milk, chicken broth, and lemon juice.

5. Stir to combine. Bring to a boil, then reduce the heat to medium-low. Simmer for 5 to 6 minutes, until the broccoli is tender.

6. Transfer the soup to a food processor and purée until smooth, or use an immersion blender.

7. Divide the soup evenly among 4 bowls. Garnish with the bacon, chives, and sliced almonds.

8. If you are preparing this dish in advance, once cool, store the soup and bacon separately in airtight containers in the refrigerator; they will keep for 4 to 5 days. Or freeze the soup in a resealable bag and defrost it in the refrigerator overnight before reheating.

Steak-lovers, this one's for you! Two kinds of mustard and a generous measure of garlic lend subtle flavor to tender top round steak in this easy broiled recipe. It's a healthy spin on a meat-lover's staple that's perfect for your busy weeknights or weekend dinner gatherings.

Ingredients:

• 2 garlic cloves, minced

• 1 Tbsp. coarse-grain Dijon mustard

• 1 Tbsp. Worcestershire sauce

• 1 tsp. ground mustard

• 1/8 tsp. salt

• 1/2 tsp. freshly ground black pepper

• 1 1/2 lb. boneless top round steak, 3/4-inch thick

Directions:

1. Heat oven to broil.

2. Whisk together garlic, Dijon mustard, Worcestershire sauce, ground mustard, salt and pepper in a small mixing bowl.

3. Line a broiler pan with foil and place steak on top. Coat evenly with mustard mixture and let stand 10 minutes. Broil steak to desired doneness, 4 minutes per side for medium-rare. Let stand 5 minutes before slicing and serving.

Getting tired of eating the same old Instant Pot recipes over and over again? Add an Italian-inspired meal to your dinner lineup that's filled with robust flavors and clean ingredients. Best of all, this Instant Pot Tuscan Soup recipe is ready to enjoy in just 20 minutes.

Ingredients:

• 1 lb. Italian chicken sausage (hot or mild), casings removed

• 1 large onion, chopped

• 3 cloves garlic, minced

• 1 tsp. dried oregano

• ½ cup sun-dried tomatoes, drained

• Salt and black pepper, to taste

• 6 cups chicken broth, low sodium

• 1 bunch kale, leaves stripped from stems and chopped

• ¾ cup heavy cream

• ¼ cup grated parmesan

• Fresh parsley, chopped (optional)

Directions:

1. Set a 6-Quart Instant Pot to sauté mode. Add the chicken sausage (casings removed) and break it up with a spoon while cooking. Continue cooking until the sausage is lightly browned, about 3-5 minutes.

2. Add in the garlic, onion and oregano. Stir constantly until the onions become translucent, about 2-3 minutes.

3. Add in the chicken broth and sun-dried tomatoes. Stir to combine. Season with pepper.

4. Set the Instant to Pot to Manual High Pressure for 5 minutes. When finished cooking, do a Quick-release.

5. Select sauté mode and add in the kale. Stir until wilted, about 1-2 minutes.

6. Stir in the heavy cream and continue cooking until heated through, about 1 minute. Season with salt and pepper to taste, as needed. Remove from the heat.

7. Garnish with fresh grated parmesan and parsley and serve immediately.

You've probably heard that breakfast is the most important meal of the day. But if you're waking up to this Steak and Egg Breakfast Bowl, it's also the most delicious. A vibrant combination of vegetables, kimchi and meat is topped with a runny egg and a dollop of smooth avocado-butter sauce for a well-balanced morning meal in a bowl.

Ingredients:

• Breakfast Bowl

• 1/2 lb. skirt steak

• 1 tsp. steak seasoning

• 3 Tbsp. avocado oil, divided

• 1 medium zucchini or yellow squash, sliced

• 6 broccolini, trimmed and cut into 2-inch pieces

• 8 small asparagus spears, trimmed and cut into 2-inch pieces

• 1/2 cup kimchi

- 1/2 avocado, sliced

- 2 scallions, thinly sliced

- 2 Tbsp. chopped cilantro

- 4 eggs

- Avocado Butter Sauce

- 1/2 ripe avocado

- 2 Tbsp. butter, room temperature

- 3 Tbsp. finely chopped fresh Italian parsley

- 1/8 tsp. cayenne pepper (optional)

- Salt and pepper, to taste

Directions:

1. Pat the steak dry, then rub with 1 tablespoon of avocado oil. Sprinkle with steak seasoning on both sides.

2. Heat 1/2 tablespoon of avocado oil in a large skillet over medium-high heat. Add the steak and cook for 3 to 4 minutes per side for medium rare. Transfer to a plate, tent with aluminum foil to keep warm, and set aside.

3. Heat another 1/2 tablespoon of avocado oil in a large skillet over medium heat. Add the zucchini, broccolini and asparagus. Cook for 2 to 3 minutes, until crisp-tender. Transfer to a plate.

4. Add the remaining 1 tablespoon of avocado oil to the pan over medium-low heat. Add the eggs and cook 3 to 5 minutes, stirring often until cooked to your preference.

5. To make the dressing, combine avocado, butter, parsley, cayenne (optional), salt and pepper in a blender or food processor. Blend until smooth.

6. Slice the steak into strips and divide among 4 serving bowls. Top with vegetables, kimchi, avocado, scallions and cilantro. Top with eggs, then drizzle with the avocado sauce. Season with salt and pepper to taste.

Brownies don't have to destroy your low carb diet! Especially when they're made with healthy ingredients like black beans. For this delicious flourless black bean brownie recipe, you'll also use chocolate protein powder to pump up the protein and chocolaty flavor.

Ingredients:

• Cooking spray

• 1 15 oz. can of black beans, no salt/sugar added

• 3 large eggs

• 3 Tbsp. canola oil or oil of choice

• 1 serving chocolate protein powder

• ½ tsp. baking soda

• ¼ tsp. salt

• 1 tsp. vanilla extract

• ¼ tsp. cinnamon

• Sugar substitute (optional, to taste)

• Water (1-2 Tbsp. as needed)

• 1 Tbsp. dark chocolate chips, sugar free, stevia sweetened

Directions:

1. Preheat oven to 350°F. Lightly grease an 8x8 baking dish with cooking spray. Note: you can use also a standard 12 slot muffin pan if you don't have a baking dish available.

2. Rinse and thoroughly drain your black beans. Combine all ingredients (except the chocolate chips) and puree in a food processor or blender until nice and smooth, scraping down the sides as needed. Note: if the batter appears too thick you can add 1-2 tablespoons of water and pulse again until a brownie batter consistency is achieved. You can also add sugar substitute (stevia or monk fruit) to taste as desired.

3. Add in chocolate chips and fold into batter. Note: you can also save the chocolate chips and sprinkle them over the top of the batter before placing the brownies in the oven.

4. Pour the batter into the baking dish (or muffin tins) and bake for about 25 to 30 minutes or until a knife inserted into the center of the brownies comes out clean.

5. Remove from the oven and let cool for at least 10 minutes before slicing your brownies into 12 evenly sliced pieces. Enjoy! Note: you can store your brownies in an airtight container for a few days or you can refrigerate them to keep even longer.

Spice up your low-carb menu with these delicious Zucchini Chicken Enchiladas. Made with a few low-carb swaps yet loaded with all of the classic enchilada flavors, these hearty Zucchini Chicken Enchiladas are the real deal. And did we mention you can enjoy them with absolutely zero guilt?!

Ingredients:

• 1 Tbsp. olive oil

• 1 large sweet onion, chopped

• 1/4 tsp. salt

• 1/4 tsp. pepper

• 2 cloves garlic, minced

• 1 tsp. ground cumin

• 2 tsp. chili powder

• 3 cups rotisserie chicken, shredded

• 1 1/2 cup red enchilada sauce, canned and divided

• 3 large zucchini — sliced thin

- 1 1/2 cup shredded Mexican cheese

- 2 avocado, diced

- 1/2 cup sour cream, for topping

- Fresh cilantro, chopped

Directions:

1. Preheat oven to 350°F.

2. Wash the zucchini. Then using a knife, mandolin or large vegetable peeler, cut the zucchini in half length-wise and then make very thin slices of the zucchini.

3. Heat a large skillet with the olive oil over medium heat. Add the chopped onion, salt and pepper.

4. Cook until translucent, about 3-5 minutes. Add the minced garlic, chicken, cumin, chili powder and 1 cup of the enchilada sauce.

5. Stir until combined and mixture is heated through.

6. On a cutting board, take 4 slices of the zucchini and overlap them slightly. Add 2 Tbsp. of the chicken mixture on top of the zucchini and then tightly roll up. Transfer to

a 9x9 baking dish with the seam facing down so the roll stays together. Repeat until the baking dish is full.

7. Top with the remaining enchilada sauce

8. Cover evenly with the shredded Mexican cheese

9. Bake for 20 minutes, until the cheese is completely melted.

10. Allow to cool for about 5 minutes and cut into 8 servings

11. Garnish with 1/4 avocado, 1 Tbsp. sour cream and fresh chopped cilantro

These are thick, fluffy, crowd-pleasing pancakes. Serve them with whipped cream, sugar-free maple syrup and a few berries for the ultimate weekend breakfast. Add a side of bacon or breakfast sausage for extra protein!

Ingredients:

• 2 large eggs

• 1/2 cup whole milk

• 1 tsp. vanilla extract

• 1 1/2 cups almond flour

• 1 tsp. baking powder

• 1/4 tsp. baking soda

• 1/8 tsp. sea salt

• 1 Tbsp. butter

• 1 cup homemade whipped cream (see link in description above)

Directions:

1. Whisk together eggs, milk and vanilla in a mixing bowl.

2. In a separate bowl, whisk together almond flour, baking powder, baking soda and salt.

3. Add dry ingredients to wet ingredients and stir well until just combined.

4. Melt 1/2 tablespoon of butter in a large pan over medium heat.

5. Drop batter into the pan, 1/4 cup at a time. Cook for 2 to 3 minutes per side, until golden.

6. Repeat with remaining butter and pancake batter until all of the pancakes are cooked.

7. Divide pancakes among 3 plates, Top with whipped cream and eat immediately.

Craving a hot, cheesy slice of pizza on your low-carb diet? Dig into these low-carb Pizza Zucchini Boats that are fully loaded with all of your favorite toppings. This low-carb take on a supreme pie is just what your Friday night needed.

Ingredients:

• 4 zucchini, sliced in half lengthwise and seeded

• 8 oz. ground Italian sausage

• 1 tsp. olive oil

• 4 oz. baby portobello mushrooms, sliced

• 1 (14-oz.) can tomato sauce

• 1 ½ cups shredded mozzarella cheese

• ½ red onion, diced

• ½ green pepper, diced

• 2 Tbsp. sliced black olives

• Fresh basil and red pepper flakes, to taste

Directions:

1. Preheat the oven to 400°F. Line a baking sheet with parchment paper. Set aside.

2. If zucchini halves don't lie flat, trim a thin strip from the bottom to create a flat surface. Arrange zucchini on the prepared baking sheet. Set aside.

3. Heat a large skillet over medium-high heat. Add sausage and cook for 4 to 6 minutes, until browned, breaking up with a wooden spoon as it cooks.

4. Heat olive oil in a small skillet over medium heat. Add mushrooms and cook for 2 to 3 minutes, until just softened.

5. Spoon 2 tablespoons of tomato sauce into each zucchini half. Top with sausage, mushrooms, mozzarella cheese, red onion, green pepper and black olives.

6. Bake for 12 to 15 minutes. Top with fresh basil and red pepper flakes before serving.

Looking for a hearty and healthy meal that the whole family will enjoy? Grab your Instant Pot and whip up this zesty taco soup for an easy dinner with minimal clean up.

Ingredients:

• 2 Tbsp. olive oil

• 1 green pepper, chopped

• ½ onion, chopped

• 3 garlic cloves, minced

• 1 ½ lb. boneless, skinless chicken breasts

• 6 cups chicken broth

• 1-10 oz. can diced tomatoes and green chilies

• 2 Tbsp. butter

• 2 Tbsp. chili seasoning

• 1 tsp. cumin

• 1 tsp. dried oregano

• 1 packet ranch seasoning mix

• 4 oz. cream cheese, softened

• Salt and pepper, to taste

Directions:

1. Set Instant Pot to sauté function and allow to heat. Add the olive oil, then the chopped green peppers, onions and garlic. Sauté, stirring constantly until the onions and green peppers begin to soften (about 3-4 minutes).

2. Pour in about ½ cup of the chicken broth, then use a wooden spoon to scrape any brown bits that may be stuck to the bottom.

3. Add the chicken to the pot and top with all of the other ingredients except for the ranch seasoning and cream cheese. Place the lid on the Instant Pot to seal.

4. Set to high pressure for 14 minutes.

5. Once the cooking time has completed, allow a 5-minute natural pressure release, then do a quick release by turning the pressure valve to release the steam.

6. Once all the steam has released, remove the lid.

7. Move the chicken breasts to a plate and shred using two forks. Set aside.

8. Turn the Instant Pot back on to the sauté function and add the ranch seasoning.

9. In a medium sized bowl, add in the softened cream cheese and about 1 cup of the soup mixture from the Instant Pot. Use an immersion blender or whisk to combine the cream cheese and soup thoroughly. Pour the mixture back into the Instant Pot. Stir to combine.

10. Boil for about 3 minutes on sauté function, then add back in the chicken. Season with salt and pepper to taste.

An Italian classic reimagined for a low-carb diet. Juicy slices of eggplant are baked in a savory almond flour coating, then smothered in homemade tomato sauce and a duo of delicious cheeses. Whip up this low carb Eggplant Parmesan for the ultimate plant-based meal.

Ingredients:

• 1 ¼ lb. eggplant

• 1 egg

• 1 Tbsp. water

• 1 cup almond flour

• 1 tsp. garlic powder

• 1 tsp. dried rosemary

• 1 tsp. dried thyme

• ½ tsp. dried oregano

• 1 cup crushed tomatoes

• 1 cup shredded mozzarella

• ¼ cup grated Parmesan

• 2 Tbsp. chopped parsley

• Olive oil spray

Directions:

1. Preheat oven to 425°F.

2. Grease a sheet pan. Set aside.

3. Trim ends from eggplant and discard. Cut remaining eggplant into ½-inch thick rounds.

4. Whisk the egg with 1 tablespoon of water in a shallow bowl.

5. Combine almond flour, garlic powder, rosemary, thyme, oregano and salt and pepper to taste in a separate shallow bowl.

6. Working in an assembly line, dip eggplant slices in egg wash and allow excess to drip away. Then press eggplant into almond meal to coat.

7. Transfer coated eggplant to the prepared baking sheet.

8. Bake eggplant for 20 minutes. Flip and bake another 10 minutes, until golden and tender.

9. Grease an 8x8 baking dish. Set aside.

10. Spray olive oil in a small pot and heat over medium. Add garlic and sauté 1 minute, until golden and fragrant.

11. Add tomatoes and bring to a boil. Reduce heat to low and simmer 4-5 minutes, until warm. Set aside.

12. Transfer enough eggplant slices to line the bottom of prepared 8x8 baking dish. Top with ½ cup tomato sauce, ½ cup mozzarella, and 2 tablespoons Parmesan. Repeat to make 2 layers.

13. Transfer baking dish to oven for 10-15 minutes, until cheese is bubbling and golden.

14. Garnish with fresh parsley before serving.

Embrace the power of cauliflower! This cruciferous veggie may seem like a bland ingredient. However, with a little creativity and a whole lot of love, you can transform it into an easy, cheesy, garlicky snack that's packed with flavor. Check out this recipe for Cheesy Garlic Cauliflower Breadsticks! It's the perfect addition to your healthy pizza or movie night and would also make a great game day appetizer.

Ingredients:

• 2 cups cauliflower rice

• ¾ cup shredded whole-milk mozzarella cheese, divided

• 6 Tbsp. grated Parmesan cheese, divided

• 1 large egg

• 3 tsp. minced garlic

• 2 Tbsp. olive oil

• 2 tsp. dried minced onion

• ½ tsp. dried thyme

- ½ tsp. dried rosemary

- ¼ tsp. dried oregano

Directions:

1. Place oven racks on the top and middle rungs of the oven and preheat it to 450°F. Line a baking sheet with parchment paper and set it aside.

2. Press the cauliflower rice between 2 clean towels to remove the excess liquid. Transfer it to a large mixing bowl.

3. Add ½ cup of the mozzarella, 4 tablespoons of the Parmesan, the egg, and the minced garlic. Season with salt and pepper to taste. Stir to combine into a dough that holds its shape when pinched together.

4. Transfer the dough to the prepared baking sheet. Press it into an oval about ¼ inch thick.

5. Transfer the baking sheet to the lower of the 2 oven racks and bake for 12 to 15 minutes, until the bottom is crisp and golden.

6. Meanwhile, whisk together in a small bowl the olive oil, minced onion, thyme, rosemary, and oregano. Season with salt and pepper to taste and set the mixture aside.

7. Remove the baking sheet from the oven. Increase the heat to broil.

8. Brush the olive oil mixture all over the bread and then sprinkle it with the remaining mozzarella and Parmesan. Return it to the top rack of the oven and broil for 1 to 2 minutes, until the cheese is bubbly and golden. Keep a close eye on the bread to prevent burning.

9. Allow the bread to cool for 5 minutes. Cut it into 12 slices and enjoy it warm.

This Hot and Cheesy Portobello Pizza recipe is the perfect solution for pizza-lovers who want to eat their pie and lose weight, too. That's because it's got all the hot and cheesy appeal of everyone's favorite takeout meal, without all the calories, sodium, fat and other general diet destruction.

Ingredients:

• 1 cup mozzarella cheese, shredded

• ½ cup spaghetti sauce, no sugar added

• 4 large portobello mushroom caps

• 2 Tbsp. nutritional yeast

• 1 Tbsp. Italian seasoning

• 5 grape tomatoes, sliced

Directions:

1. Preheat the oven to 375°F and spray a baking dish with nonstick cooking spray.

2. Place mushroom caps in the bottom of a baking dish. Spoon spaghetti sauce equally into each mushroom cap.

3. Sprinkle the mozzarella cheese, nutritional yeast and Italian seasoning equally into each mushroom cap.

4. Top each pizza with sliced tomatoes.

5. Bake for 30 minutes or until hot and bubbly.

Enjoy a guilt-free, holiday feast with our South Beach-approved Sausage Stuffing. It's low carb and absolutely delicious.

Ingredients:

• 1 loaf almond flour bread, torn or cut into 1x1 inch pieces (see separate recipe above)

• 3 Tbsp. butter, melted

• ½ lb. pork sausage

• ¾ cup celery, diced

• ¼ cup onion, minced

• 2 garlic cloves, minced

• ½ cup fresh parsley, chopped

• 2 Tbsp. fresh sage, chopped

• ½ Tbsp. fresh rosemary

• 1 Tbsp. fresh thyme

• 1 ½ cup chicken stock, low sodium

• 1 large egg

• Salt and pepper, to taste

Directions:

1. Preheat oven to 350°F and prepare a medium baking dish with cooking spray.

2. In a large bowl, lightly toss bread in melted butter. Spread evenly on a baking sheet and toast for 10 minutes.

3. Cook ground sausage in a large pan over medium heat, stirring occasionally until no longer pink (about 8-10 minutes). Season with pepper and remove sausage using a slotted spoon.

4. Add onion and celery to the pan and cook until soft, about 5 minutes.

5. Stir in garlic, parsley, sage, thyme and rosemary and continue cooking for 1 more minute. Season with salt and pepper.

6. Place toasted bread in a large bowl and add vegetable mixture and sausage. Toss lightly to combine.

7. In a small bowl, whisk together chicken broth and egg. Pour it over the bread and sausage mixture. Season with salt and pepper and toss until completely coated.

8. Transfer mixture to a baking dish and cover with foil. Bake until cooked through, about 35 minutes. Remove foil and cook for another 15 minutes until bread is crisp on top.

Check out this comfort food classic with a cheesy twist! Packed with flavor yet low in carbs, our hearty and healthy meatloaf recipe is the ultimate meat lover's dinner for your low-carb diet. The juicy blend of beef and pork is seasoned with classic Italian herbs, then stuffed with roasted red peppers, arugula and mozzarella cheese. Make it for a crowd or freeze individual slices for an easy meal prep solution.

Ingredients:

• 1 lb. ground beef

• 1/2 lb. ground pork

• 1/3 cup chopped onion

• 2 Tbsp. minced garlic

• 3 Tbsp. tomato paste

• 1/2 cup almond flour

• 2 eggs

• 1 tsp. dried rosemary

- 1 tsp. dried oregano

- 1 tsp. thyme

- 1/4 cup chopped parsley, divided

- 1/4 cup roasted red peppers, chopped

- 1 cup chopped arugula

- 1 cup shredded mozzarella

Directions:

1. Preheat oven to 375°F.

2. Line a sheet pan with parchment paper. Set aside.

3. In a large bowl, combine beef, pork, onion, garlic, tomato paste, almond flour, eggs, rosemary, oregano, thyme and half of the parsley. Add salt and pepper to taste and mix until well combined.

4. Spread the beef mixture out on the prepared baking sheet to make a large rectangle, about 1/2-inch thick.

5. Sprinkle the rectangle evenly with half of the mozzarella, roasted red peppers, arugula and remaining mozzarella, leaving a 1-inch border on the sides.

6. Using the parchment paper as a guide, roll meatloaf into a cylinder. Press seam and sides to seal.

7. Bake 45 to 55 minutes, until golden and cooked through.

8. Allow the meatloaf to rest for 10 minutes before cutting it into 8 slices.

Sweet and cinnamon-y, who doesn't love delicious Cinnamon Roll to kick off your day? The problem with this famous pastry is the loads of calories, sugar and carbs that often accompany it.

Ingredients:

• Muffins

• ½ cup almond flour

• 1 packet South Beach Diet Simply Fit Vanilla Shake Mix

• 1 tsp. baking powder

• 1 Tbsp. cinnamon

• ½ cup peanut butter

• ½ cup pumpkin puree

• ½ cup coconut oil melted (measured solid)

• Glaze

• ¼ cream cheese, softened

• ¼ cup whole milk

• 3 Tbsp. Swerve granulated sweetener

• 2 tsp. lemon juice

Directions:

1. Preheat the oven to 350 F and spray a 12 muffin tin with cooking spray or line with baking cups. Set aside.

2. In a large mixing bowl, combine the dry ingredients and mix well. Add the wet ingredients and mix until fully incorporated.

3. Distribute the muffin batter evenly in each muffin cup. Bake for about 15 minutes. The muffins are done when a toothpick comes out clean. Allow to cool in the muffin tin for about 5 minutes, before transferring to a wire rack to cool completely.

4. Once cooled, prepare your glaze by combining all ingredients and mixing until combined. Drizzle over the muffins.

Takeout and food delivery have quickly become engrained into our lives. While we can all appreciate a quick, easy and delicious dinner, there's no arguing that most fast food and restaurant meals are slim down saboteurs. Enjoy your favorite Chinese takeout order without ruining your weight loss progress with this low-carb spin on classic sesame chicken! It's filled with flavor, packed with protein and light on carbs.

Ingredients:

• 1 lb. boneless skinless chicken thighs

• 2 Tbsp. olive oil

• 2 tsp. tapioca flour

• 2 Tbsp. sesame seeds

• 1/4 cup chopped fresh cilantro

• 4 lime wedges

• Marinade

• 1/4 cup coconut aminos

- 1 tsp. erythritol brown sugar replacement

- 1 Tbsp. minced fresh garlic

- 1 Tbsp. minced fresh gingerroot

- 2 tsp. sesame oil

- 3 Tbsp. rice wine vinegar

Directions:

1. Pat the chicken dry. Dice into ½-inch pieces and season it with salt and pepper to taste.

2. In a large mixing bowl, whisk together the coconut aminos, erythritol brown sugar, garlic, ginger, sesame oil, rice wine vinegar, and salt and pepper to taste. Add the chicken and toss to coat. Cover and transfer to the refrigerator for 30 minutes to marinate.

3. Heat the olive oil over medium-high heat in a large sauté pan.

4. Remove the chicken from the marinade, allowing the excess to drip away. Reserve the marinade. Place the chicken in the hot pan and cook for 3 to 4 minutes per side.

5. Add the tapioca flour to the marinade and whisk to combine.

6. Add the marinade to the pan with the chicken and cook for 4 to 5 minutes, until the sauce thickens.

7. Evenly divide among 4 bowls and serve the chicken garnished with sesame seeds, cilantro, and lime wedges.

8. Stored in an airtight container in the refrigerator, this dish is good for 3 to 4 days.

Takeout and food delivery have quickly become engrained into our lives. While we can all appreciate a quick, easy and delicious dinner, there's no arguing that most fast food and restaurant meals are slim down saboteurs. Enjoy your favorite Chinese takeout order without ruining your weight loss progress with this low-carb spin on classic sesame chicken! It's filled with flavor, packed with protein and light on carbs.

Ingredients:

• 1 lb. boneless skinless chicken thighs

• 2 Tbsp. olive oil

• 2 tsp. tapioca flour

• 2 Tbsp. sesame seeds

• ¼ cup chopped fresh cilantro

• 4 lime wedges

• Marinade

• ¼ cup coconut aminos

• 1 tsp. erythritol brown sugar replacement

• 1 Tbsp. minced fresh garlic

• 1 Tbsp. minced fresh gingerroot

• 2 tsp. sesame oil

• 3 Tbsp. rice wine vinegar

Directions:

1. Pat the chicken dry. Dice into 1/2-inch pieces and season it with salt and pepper to taste.

2. In a large mixing bowl, whisk together the coconut aminos, erythritol brown sugar, garlic, ginger, sesame oil, rice wine vinegar, and salt and pepper to taste. Add the chicken and toss to coat. Cover and transfer to the refrigerator for 30 minutes to marinate.

3. Heat the olive oil over medium-high heat in a large sauté pan.

4. Remove the chicken from the marinade, allowing the excess to drip away. Reserve the marinade. Place the chicken in the hot pan and cook for 3 to 4 minutes per side.

5. Add the tapioca flour to the marinade and whisk to combine.

6. Add the marinade to the pan with the chicken and cook for 4 to 5 minutes, until the sauce thickens.

7. Evenly divide among 4 bowls and serve the chicken garnished with sesame seeds, cilantro, and lime wedges.

8. Stored in an airtight container in the refrigerator, this dish is good for 3 to 4 days.

This cleaned up version of your favorite takeout is the perfect family style meal to enjoy at home. Skip delivery and whip up our 15-minute Beef and Broccoli Stir Fry recipe for a wholesome, low-carb dinner that's filled with immune-boosting ingredients. Even the kiddos will love this one!

Ingredients:

• 1 lb. flat iron steak, sliced thinly against the grain

• 2 heads broccoli, cut into small florets

• ¼ cup olive or avocado oil

• 1 tsp. toasted sesame oil

• 1 tsp. fish sauce

• Marinade

• ¼ cup coconut aminos

• 1 tsp. ginger, freshly grated

• 2 cloves garlic, chopped

Directions:

1. Using a sharp knife, cut the flat iron steak into thin pieces going against the grain of the meat.

2. Place the beef, coconut aminos, ginger and garlic into a zip-top bag and shake gently to coat the steak. Marinate in the fridge for at least 1 hour.

3. Fill a large pot with water and bring it to a boil. Add the broccoli and cook for about 2 minutes. Remove from the heat and drain using a colander. Run the broccoli under cold water to stop it from cooking.

4. Remove the beef from the marinade and reserve marinade to use as the stir fry sauce.

5. Using a large wok or pan, heat oil over medium-high heat and stir fry the beef until it's browned, approximately 1-2 minutes. Remove the beef from the skillet.

6. Add the broccoli and stir fry until tender, approximately 2-3 minutes. Add the remaining marinade and cook for another 2-3 minutes.

7. Add the beef back into the wok or pan along with the fish sauce and sesame oil. Toss to evenly coat in the sauce before serving.

Muffins are the perfect breakfast. That's because they're perfectly portable so you can take them on your commute. Plus, they're super satisfying and can easily be made healthy. These wholesome, flavor-packed, high-fiber bran muffins are filled with tender pieces of pear and spiced with cinnamon.

Ingredients:

• 1 1/2 cups whole-grain pastry flour

• 1 cup wheat bran

• 2 Tbsp. granular sugar substitute

• 1 1/4 tsp. ground cinnamon

• 1 1/4 tsp. baking soda

• 1/4 tsp. salt

• 1 1/4 cups buttermilk

• 2 large eggs, lightly beaten

• 3 Tbsp. canola oil

• 1 Bosc pear, cored and cut into 1/4-inch dice

• 1 1/2 tsp. vanilla extract

Directions:

1. Heat oven to 350°F. Line a muffin tin with paper liners or lightly coat with cooking spray.

2. Combine flour, bran, sugar substitute, cinnamon, baking soda, and salt in a large mixing bowl. Combine buttermilk, eggs, oil, pear, and vanilla in another mixing bowl.

3. Make a well in the center of the dry ingredients. Add wet ingredients to dry ingredients and mix just to combine; do not over mix. Divide batter evenly into muffin cups. Bake for 20 minutes. Cool and serve.

Celery and nuts add flavor and crunch to this delectable turkey salad, while grapes add a hint of sweetness. Eat it with your favorite greens or stuff it into a whole grain pita pocket for a tasty sandwich that will fill you up without filling you out.

Ingredients:

• 1 1/2 pounds roast turkey or chicken, cut into 1/2-inch cubes

• 4 celery stalks, chopped

• 3/4 cup grapes, sliced in half

• 1/3 cup shelled salted pistachios, roughly chopped

• 1/3 cup mayonnaise

• 1/4 teaspoon salt

• 1/4 teaspoon freshly ground black pepper

Directions:

1. Combine turkey, celery, grapes, pistachios, mayonnaise, salt, and pepper in a large mixing bowl. Stir well to coat and refrigerate until ready to serve.

Beef and potatoes just got an upgrade! A homestyle classic is transformed into a Malaysian masterpiece in this hearty, low-carb dinner. Enjoy spiced morsels of tender beef served with a side of fragrant mashed roasted cauliflower. Undertones of coconut, lemongrass and turmeric peak through and make this meal shine. With winter just around the corner, this is one crowd-pleasing dish that is sure to warm you up.

Ingredients:

• Beef

• 1 medium red onion, chopped

• 1 (1-inch) piece fresh ginger, grated

• 1 small lemongrass stalk, tough outer leaves discarded and center roughly chopped

• 3 garlic cloves

• 2 Tbsp. cashew butter

• 1 tsp. ground coriander

- 1 tsp. ground cumin

- ½ tsp. chili powder

- 1 lime, juiced and zested

- 2 Tbsp. coconut oil

- 1 lb. beef stew meat, cut into strips

- ½ cup coconut milk

- Cauliflower Mash

- 1 small head cauliflower, cut into florets

- 2 Tbsp. coconut oil, melted

- ¼ teaspoon ground cardamom

- 1 teaspoon turmeric

- ¼ cup coconut cream

- To Serve

- Scallions, chopped

- Cilantro, chopped

- Lime wedges

Directions:

1. Beef

2. In a food processor, blend the onion, lemongrass, ginger, garlic, cashew butter, coriander, cumin, chili powder, lime zest, and lime juice to form a thick paste. Heat the coconut oil in a heavy bottom skillet over a medium-high heat. Add the beef and cook 3-4 minutes, stirring often until browned.

3. Add reserved paste and cook 2-3 minutes, stirring often. Add the coconut milk and bring to a boil, then reduce heat to medium-low. Cover and simmer 30-40 minutes, until the beef is very tender and most of the liquid has evaporated.

4. Cauliflower Mash

5. Preheat oven to 425°F. Toss cauliflower florets with coconut oil and salt and pepper to taste on a rimmed baking sheet. Bake 15-20 minutes, until cauliflower is golden brown. Transfer the roasted cauliflower to a large saucepan over medium heat. Mash with a potato masher.

6. Add cardamom, turmeric and coconut cream to the mashed cauliflower. Stir to combine. Cook 2-3 minutes, until heated through.

7. To Serve

8. Garnish the beef with chopped scallions and cilantro. Serve with lemon or lime wedges and a side of cauliflower mash.

CONCLUSION

The South Beach Diet, while mainly directed at weight loss, may promote certain healthy changes. Research shows that following a long-term eating plan that's rich in healthy carbohydrates and dietary fats, such as whole grains, unsaturated fats, vegetables and fruits, can improve your health. For example, eating a lower carbohydrate diet with healthy fats may improve your blood cholesterol levels.